FOURTH EDITION

AIDS TO THE EXAMINATION OF THE PERIPHERAL NERVOUS SYSTEM

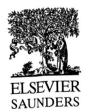

ELSEVIER
SAUNDERS

EDINBURGH · LONDON · NEW YORK · OXFORD · PHILADELPHIA · ST LOUIS · SYDNEY · TORONTO 2000

SAUNDERS
An imprint of Elsevier Limited

First published 2000
  Reprinted 2001, 2002, 2003, 2004 (twice), 2005

ISBN 0 7020 2512 7

Cataloguing in Publication Data:
Catalogue record for this book is available from the British Library and the US Library of Congress.

Library of Congress Cataloguing in Publication Data
A catalogue record for this book is available from the Library of Congress

ELSEVIER your source for books,
journals and multimedia
in the health sciences

www.elsevierhealth.com

Working together to grow
libraries in developing countries
www.elsevier.com | www.bookaid.org | www.sabre.org

ELSEVIER BOOKAID International Sabre Foundation

Printed in China
C/07

Commissioning Editor: Michael Parkinson
Project Development Manager: Sarah Keer-Keer
Project Manager: Frances Affleck
Designer: Judith Wright

PREFACE

In 1940 Dr George Riddoch was Consultant Neurologist to the Army. He realised the necessity of providing centres to deal with peripheral nerve injuries during the war. In collaboration with Professor J. R. Learmonth, Professor of Surgery at the University of Edinburgh, peripheral nerve injury centres were established at Gogarburn near Edinburgh and at Killearn near Glasgow. Professor Learmonth wished to have an illustrated guide on peripheral nerve injuries for the use of surgeons working in general hospitals. In collaboration with Dr Ritchie Russell, a few photographs demonstrating the testing of individual muscles were taken in 1941. Dr Ritchie Russell returned to Oxford in 1942 and was replaced by Dr M. J. McArdle as Neurologist to Scottish Command. The photographs were completed by Dr McArdle at Gogarburn with the help of the Department of Medical Illustration at the University of Edinburgh. About twenty copies in loose-leaf form were circulated to surgeons in Scotland.

In 1943 Professor Learmonth and Dr Riddoch added the diagrams illustrating the innervation of muscles by various peripheral nerves modified from Pitres and Testut, (*Les Neufs en Schemas*, Doin, Paris, 1925) and also the diagrams of cutaneous sensory distributions and dermatomes. This work was published by the Medical Research Council in 1943 as *Aids to the Investigation of Peripheral Nerve Injuries* (War Memorandum No. 7). It became a standard work and over the next thirty years many thousands of copies were printed.

It was thoroughly revised between 1972 and 1975 with new photographs and many new diagrams and was republished under the title *Aids to the Examination of the Peripheral Nervous System* (Memorandum No. 45), reflecting the wide use made of this booklet by students and practitioners and its more extensive use in clinical neurology, which was rather different from the war time emphasis on nerve injuries.

In 1984 the Medical Research Council transferred responsibility for this publication to the Guarantors of *Brain* for whom a new edition was prepared. Modifications were made to some of the diagrams and a new diagram of the lumbosacral plexus was included.

Most of the photographs for the 1943, 1975 and 1986 editions show Dr McArdle, who died in 1989, as the examining physician. A new set of colour photographs has been prepared for this edition, the diagrams of the brachial plexus and lumbosacral plexus have been retained, but all the other diagrams have been redrawn.

ACKNOWLEDGEMENTS

The Guarantors of *Brain* are very grateful to:

Patricia Archer PhD for the drawings of the brachial plexus and lumbosacral plexus

Ralph Hutchings for the photography

Paul Richardson for the artwork and diagrams

Michael Hutchinson MB BDS for advice on the neuro-anatomy

Sarah Keer-Keer (Harcourt Publishers) for her help and encouragement.

CONTENTS

INTRODUCTION

This atlas is intended as a guide to the examination of patients with lesions of peripheral nerves and nerve roots.

These examinations should, if possible, be conducted in a quiet room where patient and examiner will be free from distraction. For both motor and sensory testing it is important that the patient should first be warm. The nature and object of the tests should be explained to the patient so that his interest and co-operation are secured. If either shows signs of fatigue, the session should be discontinued and resumed later.

Motor testing

A muscle may act as a *prime mover,* as a *fixator,* as an *antagonist,* or as a *synergist.* Thus, flexor carpi ulnaris acts as a *prime mover* when it flexes and adducts the wrist; as a *fixator* when it immobilises the pisiform bone during contraction of the adductor digiti minimi; as an *antagonist* when it resists extension of the wrist; and as a *synergist* when the digits, but not the wrists, are extended.

As far as possible the action of each muscle should be observed separately and a note made of those in which power has been retained as well as of those that are weak or paralysed. It is usual to examine the power of a muscle in relation to the movement of a single joint. It has long been customary to use a 0 to 5 scale for recording muscle power, but it is generally recognised that subdivision of grade 4 may be helpful.

0   No contraction
1   Flicker or trace of contraction
2   Active movement, with gravity eliminated
3   Active movement against gravity
4   Active movement against gravity and resistance
5   Normal power

Grades 4−, 4 and 4+, may be used to indicate movement against slight, moderate and strong resistance respectively.

The models employed in this work were not chosen because they showed unusual muscular development; the ease with which the contraction of muscles is identified varies with the build of the patient, and it is essential that the examiner should both look for and endeavour to feel the contraction of an accessible muscle and/or the movement of its tendon. In most of the illustrations the optimum point for palpation has been marked.

Muscles have been arranged in the order of the origin of their motor supply from nerve trunks, which is convenient in many examinations. Usually only one method of testing each muscle is shown but, where necessary, multiple illustrations have been included if a muscle has more than one important action. The examiner should apply the tests as they are illustrated, because the techniques shown will eliminate many of the traps for the inexperienced provided by 'trick' movements. It should be noted that each of the methods used tests, as a rule, the action of muscles at a single joint.

When testing a movement, the limb should be firmly supported proximal to the relevant joint, so that the test is confined to the chosen muscle group and does not require the patient to fix the limb proximally by muscle contraction. In this book, this principle is illustrated in Figs 12, 18, 28b, 31 and many others. In some illustrations, the examiners supporting hand has been omitted for clarity (for example Figs 30, 34, 48 and 53).

The usual nerve supply to each muscle is stated in the captions, and the spinal segments from which it is derived, the more important of the latter being printed in heavy type. Tables showing limb muscles arranged according to their supply by individual nerve roots and peripheral nerves are to be found on pages 60–61.

A table showing commonly tested movements is on page 62.

Sensory testing

The patient is first asked to outline the area of sensory abnormality; this can be a useful guide to the detailed examination. Light touch should be tested by touches with something soft such as cotton wool or a light finger touch, working from the insensitive towards the normal area. If the area of sensory abnormality is hypersensitive the direction is reversed. For testing superficial pain a sharp pin should be used and again – unless there is apparent hypersensitivity (hyperpathia) – the stimuli are applied first to the analgesic area, working outwards.

It may also be important to test two-point discrimination on the fingers, joint position sense and, on occasion, deep pressure sense.

The area of skin supplied by any one nerve or nerve root varies from patient to patient, peripheral nerve distribution is more reliable and consistent than nerve root supply. The areas shown in the diagrams are the usual ones.

SPINAL ACCESSORY NERVE

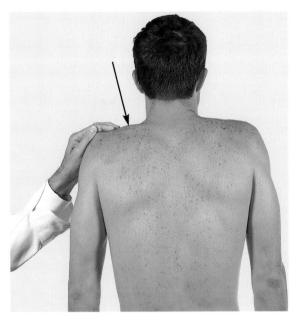

Fig. 1 Trapezius (Spinal accessory nerve and C3, C4)

The patient is elevating the shoulder against resistance.
Arrow: the thick upper part of the muscle can be seen and felt.

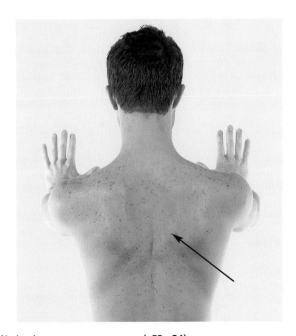

Fig. 2 Trapezius (Spinal accessory nerve and C3, C4)

The patient is pushing the palms of the hands hard against a wall with the elbows fully extended. *Arrow:* the lower fibres of trapezius can be seen and felt.

BRACHIAL PLEXUS

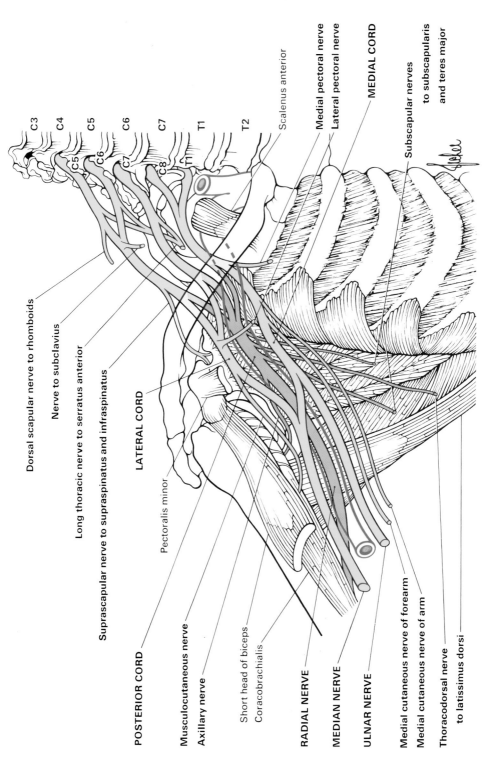

Fig. 3 Diagram of the brachial plexus, its branches and the muscles which they supply.

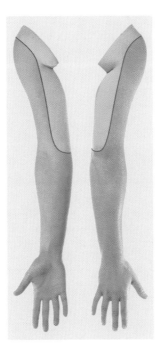

Fig. 4 The approximate area within which sensory changes may be found in complete lesions of the brachial plexus (C5, C6, C7, C8, T1).

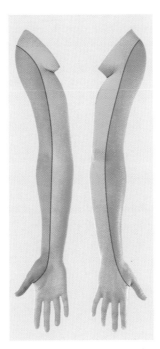

Fig. 5 The approximate area within which sensory changes may be found in lesions of the upper roots (C5,C6) of the brachial plexus.

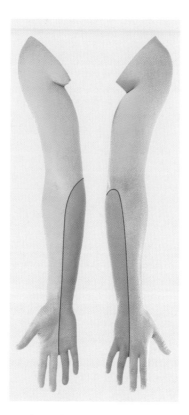

Fig. 6   The approximate area within which sensory changes may be found in lesions of the lower roots (C8, T1) of the brachial plexus.

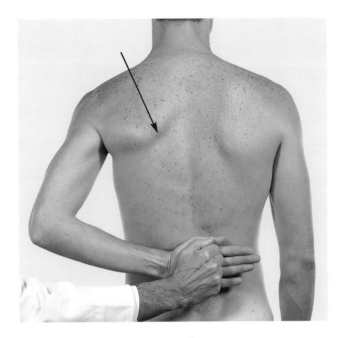

Fig. 7 Rhomboids (Dorsal scapular nerve; C4, C5)

The patient is pressing the palm of his hand backwards against the examiner's hand. *Arrow:* the muscle bellies can be felt and sometimes seen.

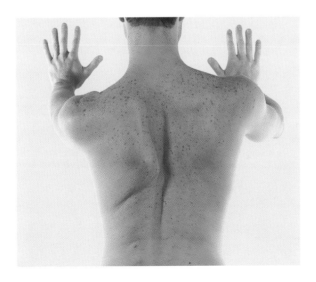

Fig. 8 Serratus anterior (Long thoracic nerve; C5, C6, C7)

The patient is pushing against a wall. The left serratus anterior is paralysed and there is winging of the scapula.

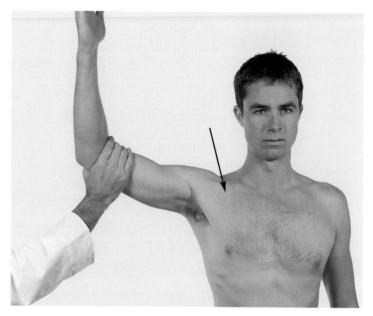

Fig. 9 Pectoralis Major: Clavicular Head (Lateral pectoral nerve; **C5**, C6)

The upper arm is above the horizontal and the patient is pushing forward against the examiner's hand. *Arrow:* the clavicular head of pectoralis major can be seen and felt.

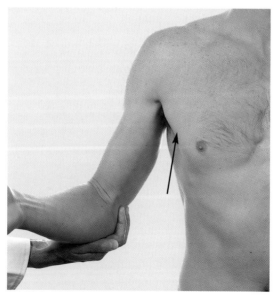

Fig. 10 Pectoralis Major: Sternocostal Head (Lateral and medial pectoral nerves; C6, **C7**, C8)

The patient is adducting the upper arm against resistance.
Arrow: the sterno-costal head can be seen and felt.

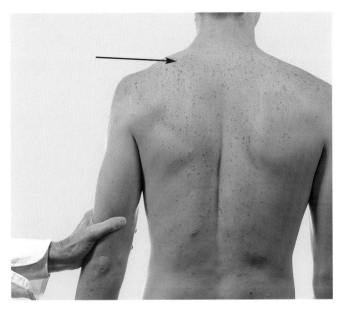

Fig. 11 Supraspinatus (Suprascapular nerve; **C5**, C6)

The patient is abducting the upper arm against resistance.
Arrow: the muscle belly can be felt and sometimes seen.

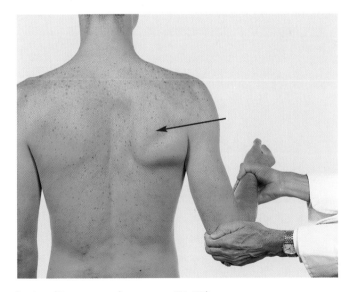

Fig. 12 Infraspinatus (Suprascapular nerve; **C5**, C6)

The patient is externally rotating the upper arm at the shoulder against resistance. The examiner's right hand is resisting the movement and supporting the forearm with the elbow at a right angle; his left hand is supporting the elbow and preventing abduction of the arm. *Arrow*: the muscle belly can be seen and felt.

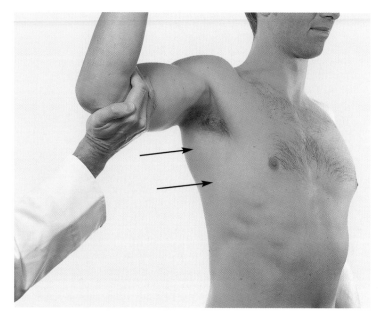

Fig. 13 Latissimus Dorsi (Thoracodorsal nerve; C6, **C7**, C8)

The upper arm is horizontal and the patient is adducting it against resistance. *Lower arrow:* the muscle belly can be seen and felt. The *upper arrow* points to teres major.

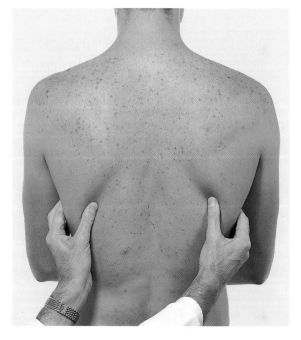

Fig. 14 Latissimus Dorsi (Thoracodorsal nerve; C6, **C7**, C8)

The Muscle bellies can be felt to contract when the patient coughs.

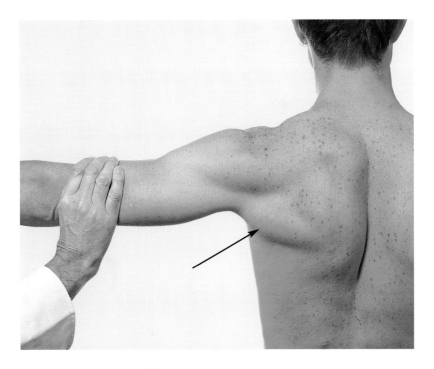

Fig. 15   Teres Major (Subscapular nerve; C5, C6, C7)
The patient is adducting the elevated upper arm against resistance.
Arrow: the muscle belly can be seen and felt.

MUSCULOCUTANEOUS NERVE

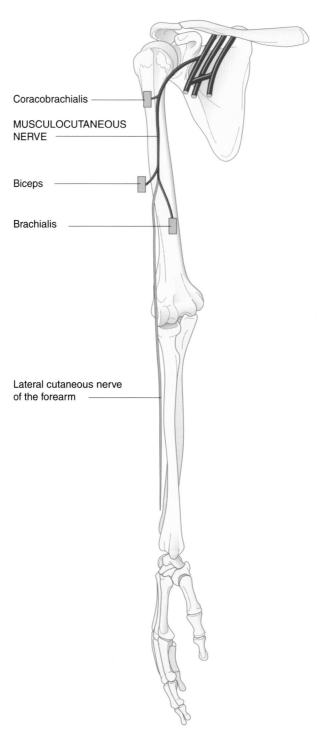

Coracobrachialis

MUSCULOCUTANEOUS
NERVE

Biceps

Brachialis

Lateral cutaneous nerve
of the forearm

Fig. 16 Diagram of the musculocutaneous nerve, its major cutaneous branch and the muscles which it supplies.

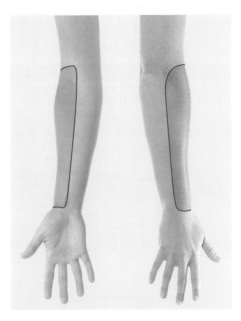

Fig. 17 The approximate area within which sensory changes may be found in lesions of the musculocutaneous nerve. (The distribution of the lateral cutaneous nerve of the forearm.)

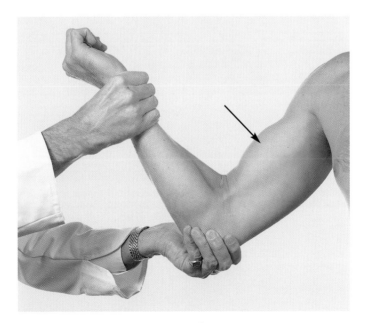

Fig. 18 Biceps (Musculocutaneous nerve; C5, C6)

The patient is flexing the supinated forearm against resistance.
Arrow: the muscle belly can be seen and felt.

AXILLARY NERVE

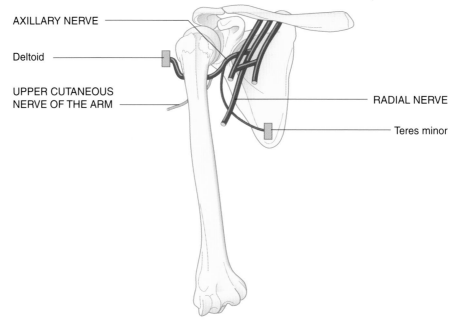

AXILLARY NERVE

Deltoid

UPPER CUTANEOUS
NERVE OF THE ARM

RADIAL NERVE

Teres minor

Fig. 19 Diagram of the axillary nerve, its major cutaneous branch and the muscles which it supplies.

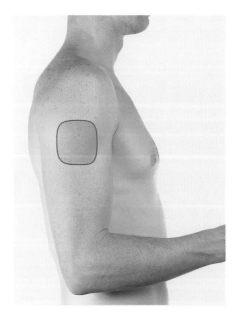

Fig. 20 The approximate area within which sensory changes may be found in lesions of the axillary nerve.

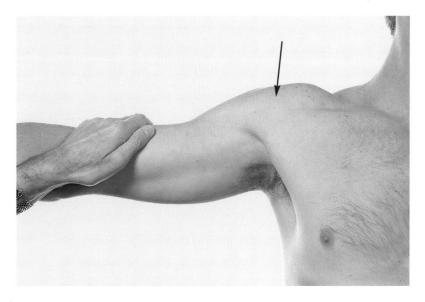

Fig. 21 Deltoid (Axillary nerve; **C5**, C6)

The patient is abducting the upper arm against resistance.
Arrow: the anterior and middle fibres of the muscle can be seen and felt.

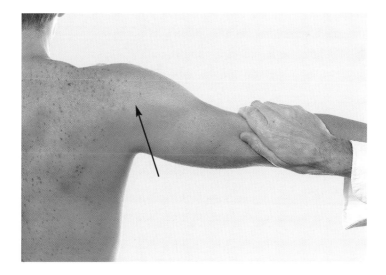

Fig. 22 Deltoid (Axillary nerve; **C5**, C6)

The patient is retracting the abducted upper arm against resistance.
Arrow: the posterior fibres of deltoid can be seen and felt.

RADIAL NERVE

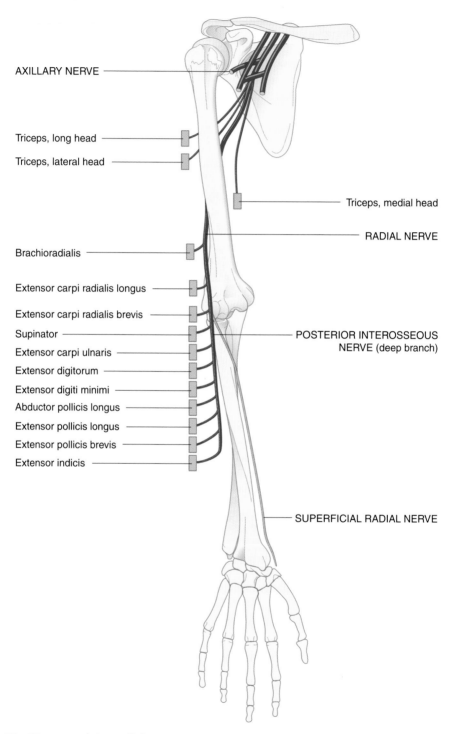

AXILLARY NERVE

Triceps, long head

Triceps, lateral head

Triceps, medial head

RADIAL NERVE

Brachioradialis

Extensor carpi radialis longus

Extensor carpi radialis brevis

Supinator

Extensor carpi ulnaris

Extensor digitorum

Extensor digiti minimi

Abductor pollicis longus

Extensor pollicis longus

Extensor pollicis brevis

Extensor indicis

POSTERIOR INTEROSSEOUS NERVE (deep branch)

SUPERFICIAL RADIAL NERVE

Fig. 23 Diagram of the radial nerve, its major cutaneous branch and the muscles which it supplies.

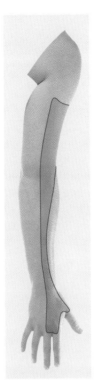

Fig. 24 The approximate area within which sensory changes may be found in high lesions of the radial nerve (above the origin of the posterior cutaneous nerves of the arm and forearm). The average area is usually considerably smaller, and absence of sensory changes has been recorded.

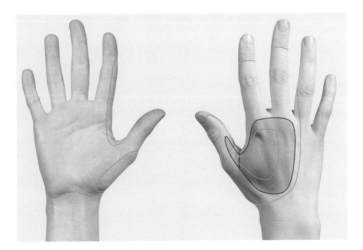

Fig. 25 The approximate area within which sensory changes may be found in lesions of the radial nerve above the elbow joint and below the origin of the posterior cutaneous nerve of the forearm. (The distribution of the superficial terminal branch of the radial nerve.) Usual area shaded, with dark blue line; light blue lines show small and large areas.

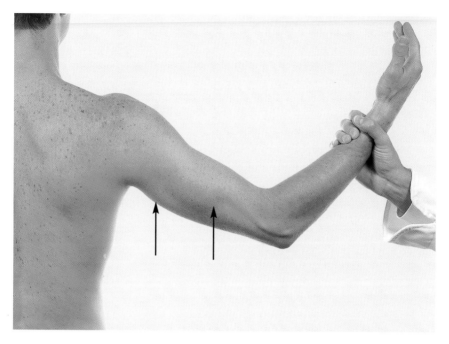

Fig. 26 Triceps (Radial nerve; C6, **C7**, C8)

The patient is extending the forearm at the elbow against resistance.
Arrows: the long and lateral heads of the muscle can be seen and felt.

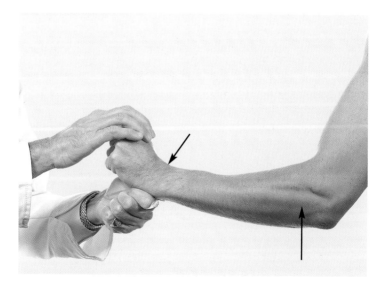

Fig. 27 Extensor Carpi Radialis Longus (Radial nerve; C5, **C6**)

The patient is extending and abducting the hand at the wrist against resistance.
Arrows: the muscle belly and tendon can be felt and usually seen.

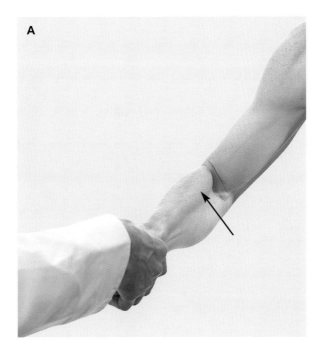

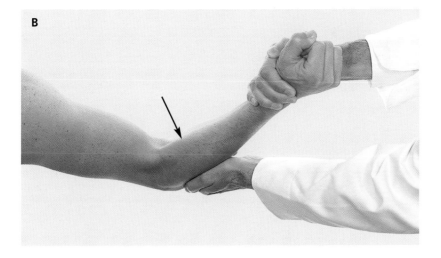

Fig. 28 Brachioradialis (Radial nerve; C5, **C6**)

The patient is flexing the forearm against resistance with the forearm midway between pronation and supination. *Arrow:* the muscle belly can be seen and felt.

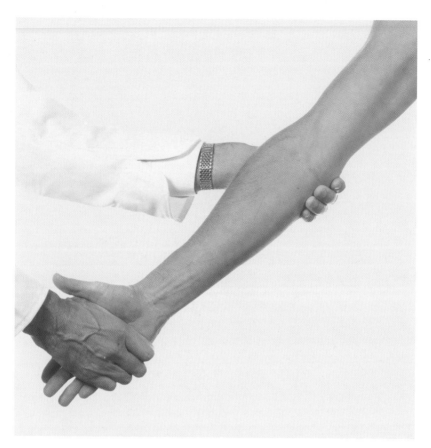

Fig. 29   Supinator (Radial nerve; C6, C7)

The patient is supinating the forearm against resistance with the forearm extended at the elbow.

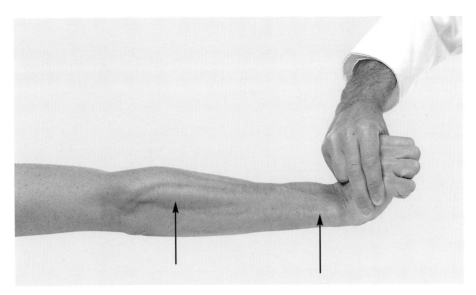

Fig. 30 Extensor Carpi Ulnaris (Posterior interosseous nerve; **C7**, C8)

The patient is extending and adducting the hand at the wrist against resistance. *Arrows*: the muscle belly and the tendon can be seen and felt.

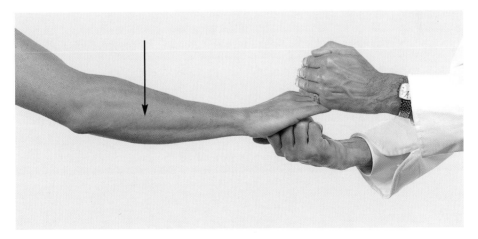

Fig. 31 Extensor Digitorum (Posterior interosseous nerve; **C7**, C8)

The patient's hand is firmly supported by the examiner's right hand. Extension at the metacarpophalangeal joints is maintained against the resistance of the fingers of the examiner's left hand. *Arrow*: the muscle belly can be seen and felt.

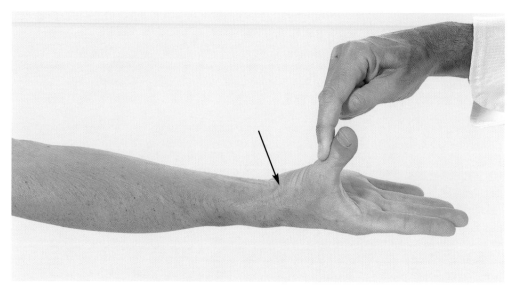

Fig. 32 Abductor Pollicis Longus (Posterior interosseous nerve; **C7**, C8)

The patient is abducting the thumb at the carpo-metacarpal joint in a plane at right angles to the palm. *Arrow*: the tendon can be seen and felt anterior and closely adjacent to the tendon of extensor pollicis brevis (**cf**. Fig. 34).

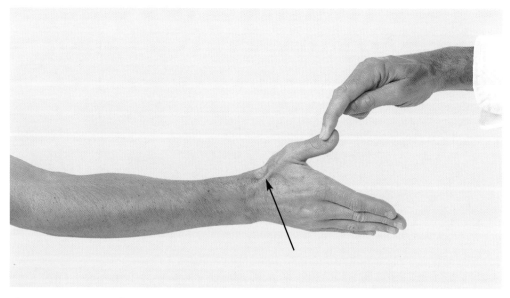

Fig. 33 Extensor Pollicis Longus (Posterior interosseous nerve; **C7**, C8)

The patient is extending the thumb at the interphalangeal joint against resistance. *Arrow*: the tendon can be seen and felt.

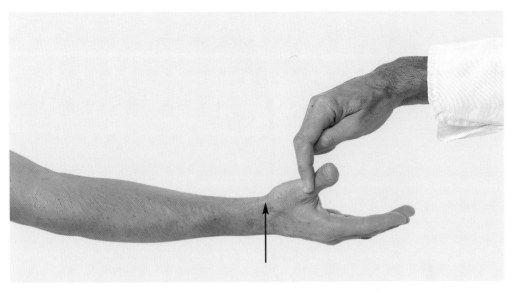

Fig. 34 Extensor Pollicis Brevis (Posterior interosseous nerve; **C7**, C8)

The patient is extending the thumb at the metacarpophalangeal joint against resistance. *Arrow*: the tendon can be seen and felt (**cf**. Fig. 32).

MEDIAN NERVE

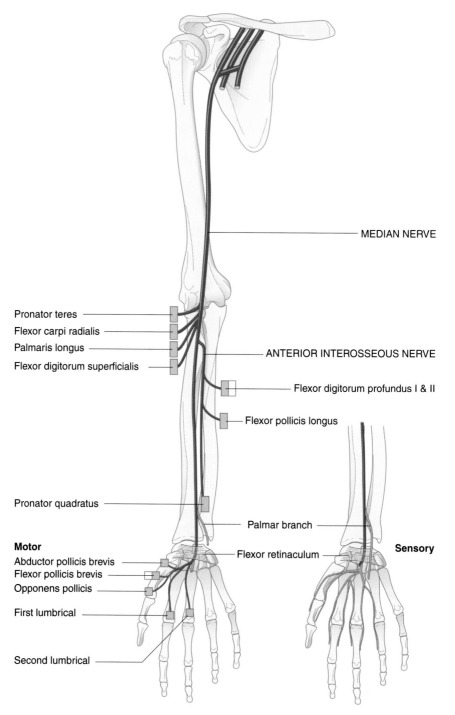

MEDIAN NERVE

Pronator teres

Flexor carpi radialis

Palmaris longus

Flexor digitorum superficialis

ANTERIOR INTEROSSEOUS NERVE

Flexor digitorum profundus I & II

Flexor pollicis longus

Pronator quadratus

Palmar branch

Motor

Sensory

Flexor retinaculum

Abductor pollicis brevis

Flexor pollicis brevis

Opponens pollicis

First lumbrical

Second lumbrical

Fig. 35 Diagram of the median nerve, its cutaneous branches and the muscles which it supplies. Note: the white rectangle signifies that the muscle indicated receives a part of its nerve supply from another peripheral nerve (**cf**. Figs. 45, 57 and 58).

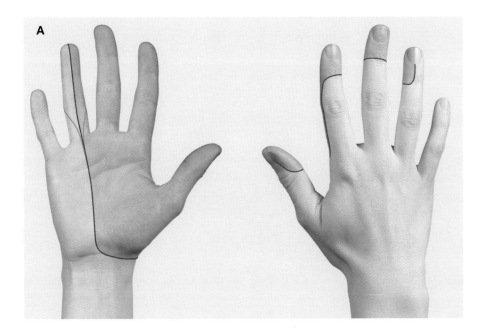

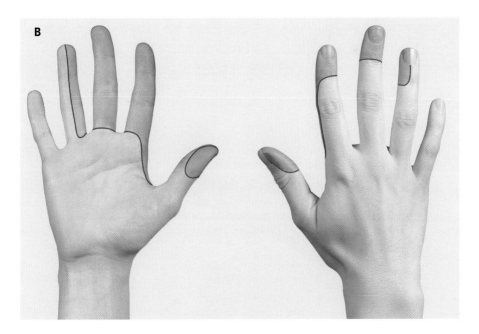

Fig. 36 The approximate areas within which sensory changes may be found in lesions of the median nerve in: **A** the forearm, **B** the carpal tunnel.

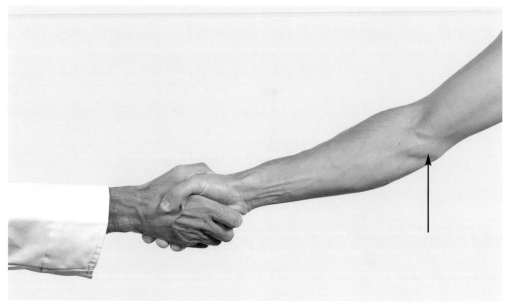

Fig. 37 Pronator Teres (Median nerve; C6, C7)

The patient is pronating the forearm against resistance.
Arrow: the muscle belly can be felt and sometime seen.

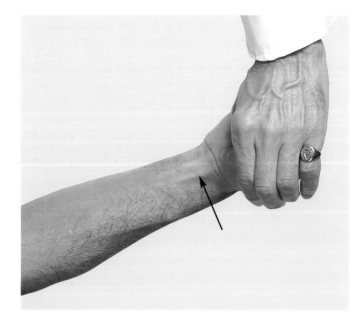

Fig. 38 Flexor Carpi Radialis (Median nerve; C6, C7)

The patient is flexing and abducting the hand at the wrist against resistance.
Arrow: the tendon can be seen and felt.

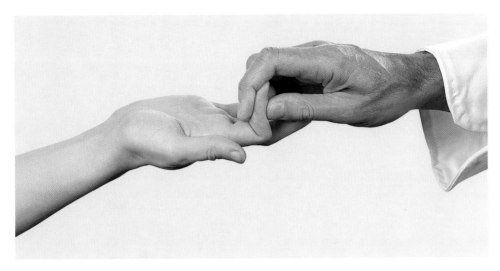

Fig. 39 Flexor Digitorum Superficialis (Median nerve; C7, **C8**, T1)

The patient is flexing the finger at the proximal interphalageal joint against resistance with the proximal phalanx fixed. This test does not eliminate the possibility of flexion at the proximal interphalangeal joint being produced by flexor digitorum profundus.

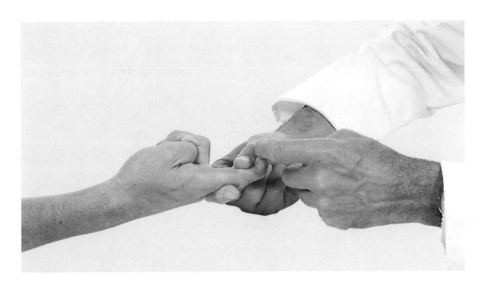

Fig. 40 Flexor Digitorum Profundus I and II (Anterior interosseous nerve; C7, **C8**)

The patient is flexing the distal phalanx of the index finger against resistance with the middle phalanx fixed.

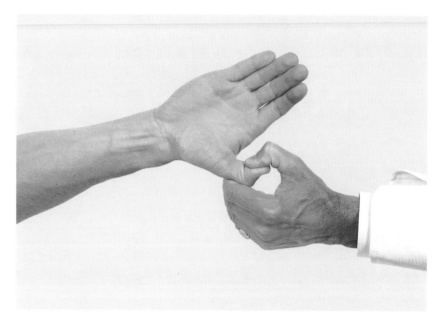

Fig. 41 Flexor Pollicis Longus (Anterior interosseous nerve; C7, **C8**)

The patient is flexing the distal phalanx of the thumb against resistance while the proximal phalanx is fixed.

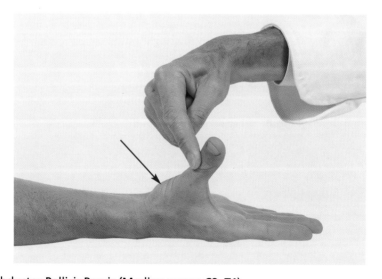

Fig. 42 Abductor Pollicis Brevis (Median nerve; C8, **T1**)

The patient is abducting the thumb at right angles to the palm against resistance. *Arrow*: the muscle can be seen and felt.

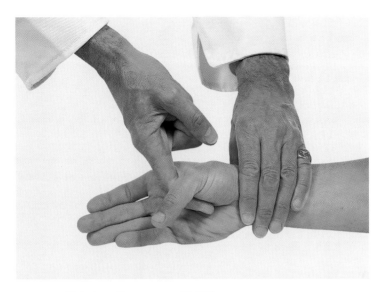

Fig. 43   Opponens Pollicis (Median nerve; C8, **T1**)

The patient is touching the base of the little finger with the thumb against resistance.

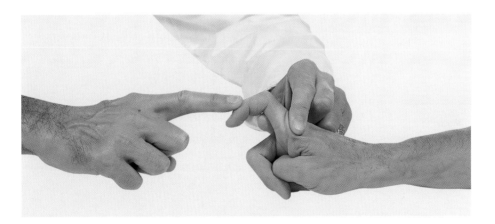

Fig. 44   1st Lumbrical-Interosseous Muscle (Median and ulnar nerves; C8, **T1**)

The patient is extending the finger at the proximal interphalangeal joint against resistance with the metacarpophalangeal joint hyperextended and fixed.

ULNAR NERVE

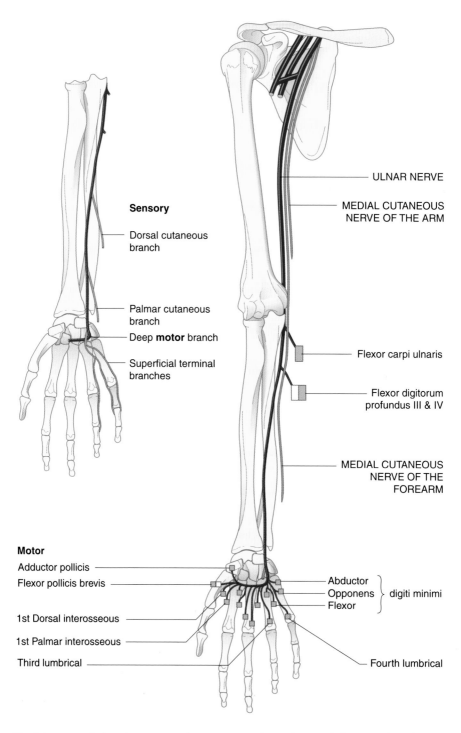

Sensory

Dorsal cutaneous branch

Palmar cutaneous branch

Deep **motor** branch

Superficial terminal branches

ULNAR NERVE

MEDIAL CUTANEOUS NERVE OF THE ARM

Flexor carpi ulnaris

Flexor digitorum profundus III & IV

MEDIAL CUTANEOUS NERVE OF THE FOREARM

Motor

Adductor pollicis

Flexor pollicis brevis

1st Dorsal interosseous

1st Palmar interosseous

Third lumbrical

Abductor
Opponens } digiti minimi
Flexor

Fourth lumbrical

Fig. 45 Diagram of the ulnar nerve, its cutaneous branches and the muscles which it supplies.

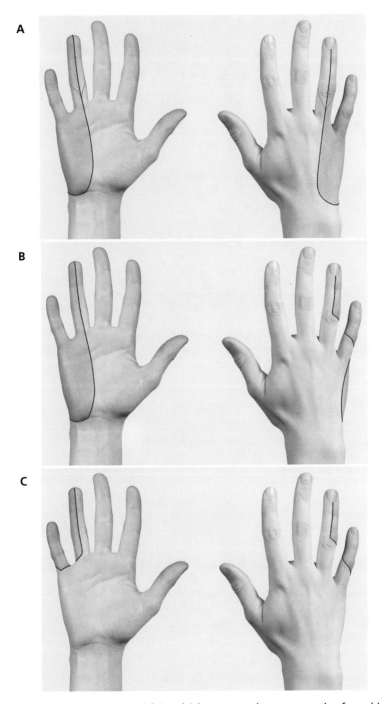

Fig. 46 The approximate areas within which sensory changes may be found in lesions of the ulnar nerve: **A** above the origin of the dorsal cutaneous branch, **B** below the origin of the dorsal cutaneous branch and above the origin of the palmar branch, **C** below the origin of the palmar branch.

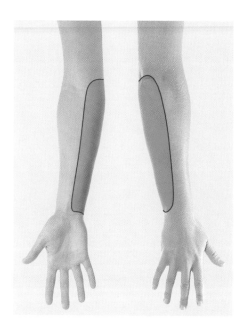

Fig. 47 The approximate area within which sensory changes may be found in lesions of the medial cutaneous nerve of the forearm.

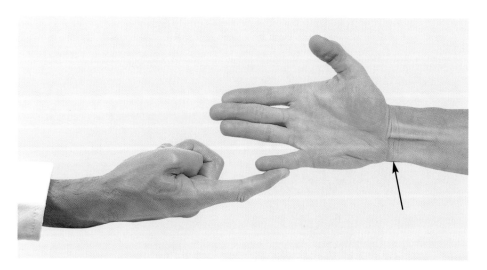

Fig. 48 Flexor Carpi Ulnaris (Ulnar nerve; C7, **C8**, T1)

The patient is abducting the little finger against resistance. The tendon of flexor carpi ulnaris can be seen and felt (*arrow*) as the muscle comes into action to fix the pisiform bone from which abductor digiti minimi arises. If flexor carpi ulnaris is intact, the tendon is seen even when abductor digiti minimi is paralysed (see also Fig. 49).

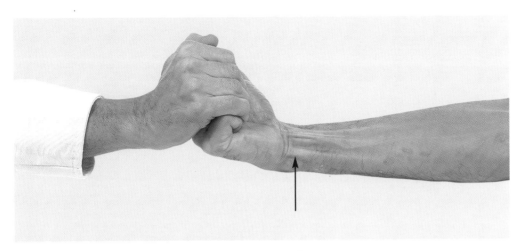

Fig. 49 Flexor Carpi Ulnaris (Ulnar nerve; C7, **C8**, T1)

The patient is flexing and adducting the hand at the wrist against resistance.
Arrow: the tendon can be seen and felt.

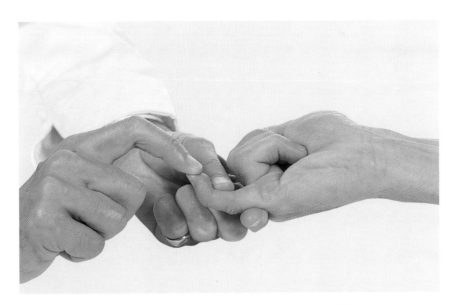

Fig. 50 Flexor Digitorum Profundus III and IV (Ulnar nerve; C7, **C8**)

The patient is flexing the distal interphalangeal joint against resistance while the middle phalanx is fixed.

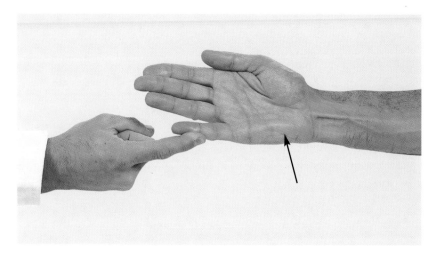

Fig. 51 Abductor Digiti Minimi (Ulnar nerve; **C8, T1**)

The patient is abducting the little finger against resistance.
Arrow: the muscle belly can be felt and seen.

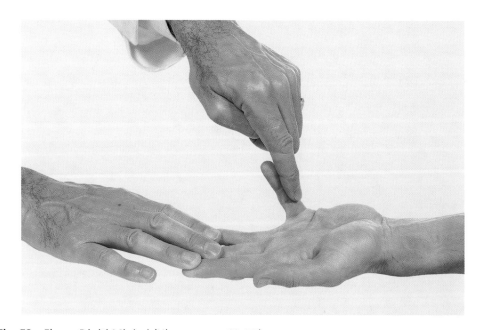

Fig. 52 Flexor Digiti Minimi (Ulnar nerve; C8, **T1**)

The patient is flexing the little finger at the metacarpophalangeal joint against resistance with the finger extended at both interphalangeal joints.

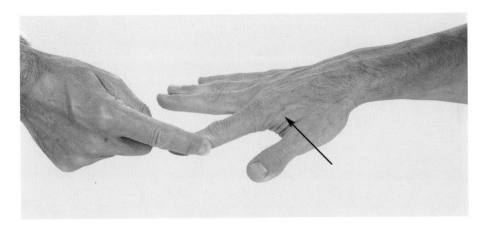

Fig. 53   First Dorsal Interosseous Muscle (Ulnar nerve; C8, **T1**)
The patient is abducting the index finger against resistance.
Arrow: the muscle belly can be felt and usually seen.

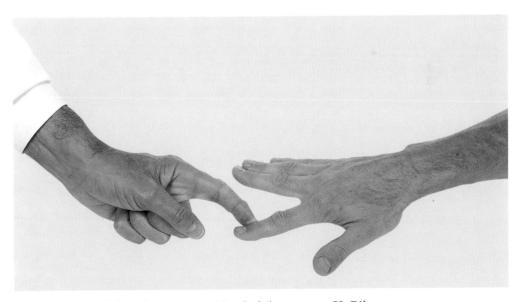

Fig. 54   Second Palmar Interosseous Muscle (Ulnar nerve; C8, **T1**)
The patient is adducting the index finger against resistance.

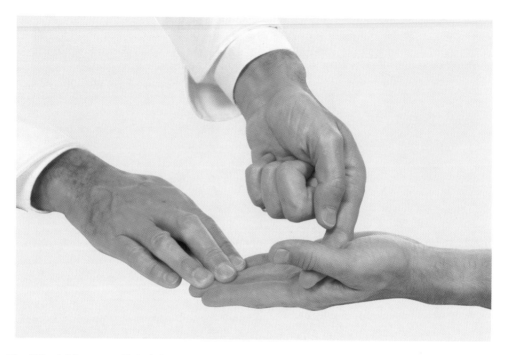

Fig. 55 Adductor Pollicis (Ulnar nerve; C8, **T1**)

The patient is adducting the thumb at right angles to the palm against the resistance of the examiner's finger.

LUMBOSACRAL PLEXUS

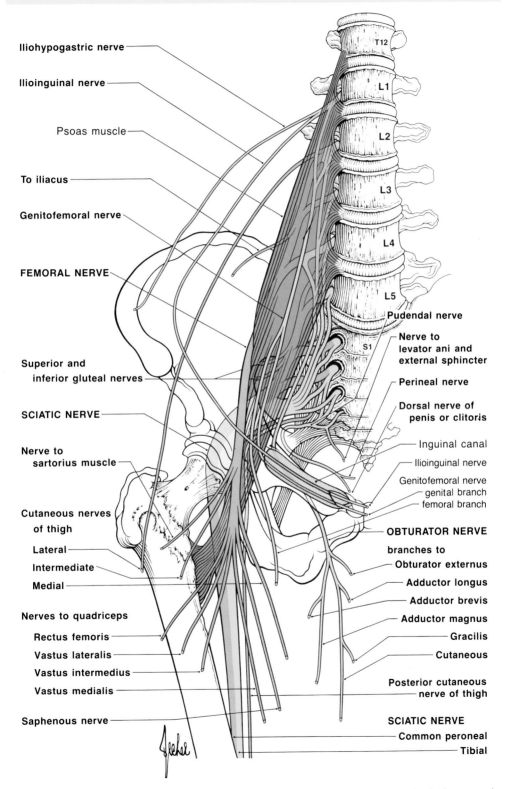

Iliohypogastric nerve

Ilioinguinal nerve

Psoas muscle

To iliacus

Genitofemoral nerve

FEMORAL NERVE

Superior and inferior gluteal nerves

SCIATIC NERVE

Nerve to sartorius muscle

Cutaneous nerves of thigh

Lateral

Intermediate

Medial

Nerves to quadriceps

Rectus femoris

Vastus lateralis

Vastus intermedius

Vastus medialis

Saphenous nerve

T12

L1

L2

L3

L4

L5

S1

Pudendal nerve

Nerve to levator ani and external sphincter

Perineal nerve

Dorsal nerve of penis or clitoris

Inguinal canal

Ilioinguinal nerve

Genitofemoral nerve
genital branch
femoral branch

OBTURATOR NERVE

branches to

Obturator externus

Adductor longus

Adductor brevis

Adductor magnus

Gracilis

Cutaneous

Posterior cutaneous nerve of thigh

SCIATIC NERVE

Common peroneal

Tibial

Fig. 56 Diagram of the lumbosacral plexus, its branches and the muscles which they supply.

NERVES OF THE LOWER LIMB

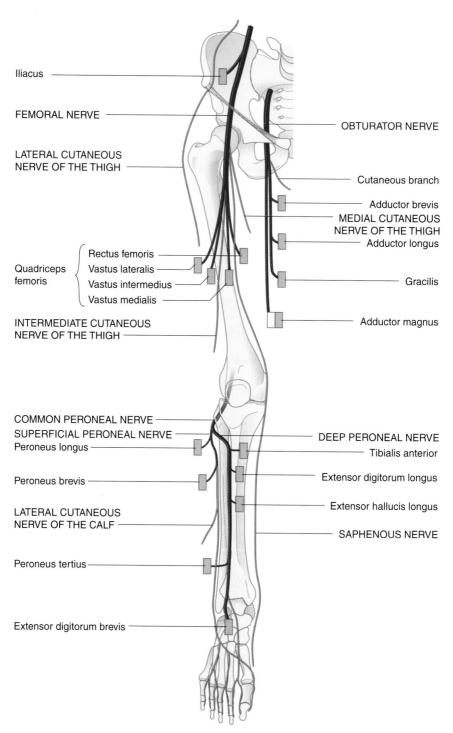

Iliacus

FEMORAL NERVE

LATERAL CUTANEOUS
NERVE OF THE THIGH

OBTURATOR NERVE

Cutaneous branch

Adductor brevis
MEDIAL CUTANEOUS
NERVE OF THE THIGH
Adductor longus

Quadriceps
femoris
{ Rectus femoris
Vastus lateralis
Vastus intermedius
Vastus medialis

Gracilis

INTERMEDIATE CUTANEOUS
NERVE OF THE THIGH

Adductor magnus

COMMON PERONEAL NERVE
SUPERFICIAL PERONEAL NERVE
Peroneus longus

DEEP PERONEAL NERVE
Tibialis anterior

Peroneus brevis

Extensor digitorum longus

Extensor hallucis longus

LATERAL CUTANEOUS
NERVE OF THE CALF

SAPHENOUS NERVE

Peroneus tertius

Extensor digitorum brevis

Fig. 57   Diagram of the nerves on the anterior aspect of the lower limb, their cutaneous branches and the muscles which they supply.

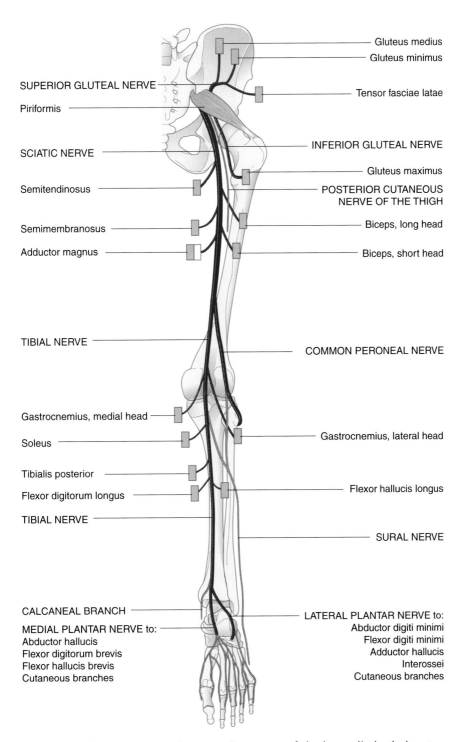

SUPERIOR GLUTEAL NERVE

Piriformis

SCIATIC NERVE

Semitendinosus

Semimembranosus

Adductor magnus

TIBIAL NERVE

Gastrocnemius, medial head

Soleus

Tibialis posterior

Flexor digitorum longus

TIBIAL NERVE

CALCANEAL BRANCH

MEDIAL PLANTAR NERVE to:
Abductor hallucis
Flexor digitorum brevis
Flexor hallucis brevis
Cutaneous branches

Gluteus medius
Gluteus minimus

Tensor fasciae latae

INFERIOR GLUTEAL NERVE

Gluteus maximus

POSTERIOR CUTANEOUS
NERVE OF THE THIGH

Biceps, long head

Biceps, short head

COMMON PERONEAL NERVE

Gastrocnemius, lateral head

Flexor hallucis longus

SURAL NERVE

LATERAL PLANTAR NERVE to:
Abductor digiti minimi
Flexor digiti minimi
Adductor hallucis
Interossei
Cutaneous branches

Fig. 58 Diagram of the nerves on the posterior aspect of the lower limb, their cutaneous branches and the muscles which they supply.

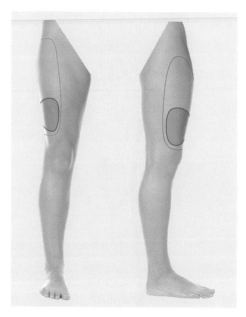

Fig. 59 The approximate area within which sensory changes may be found in lesions of the lateral cutaneous nerve of the thigh. Usual area shaded, with dark blue line; large area indicated with light blue line.

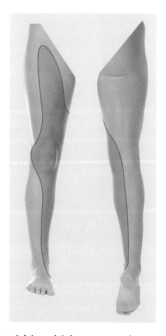

Fig. 60 The approximate area within which sensory changes may be found in lesions of the femoral nerve. (The distribution of the intermediate and medial cutaneous nerves of the thigh and the saphenous nerve.)

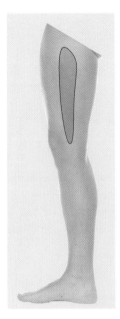

Fig. 61 The approximate area within which sensory changes may be found in lesions of the obturator nerve.

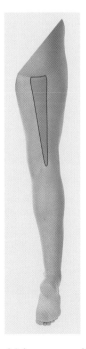

Fig. 62 The approximate area within which sensory changes may be found in lesions of the posterior cutaneous nerve of the thigh.

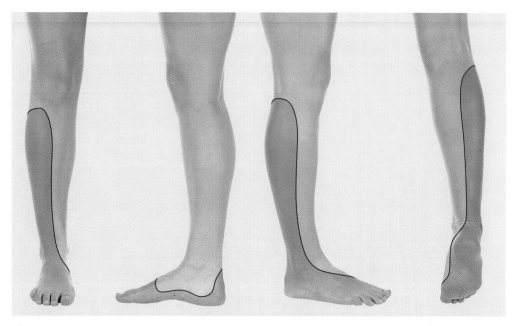

Fig. 63   The approximate area within which sensory changes may be found in lesions of the trunk of the sciatic nerve. (Modified from M.R.C. Special Report No. 54, 1920.)

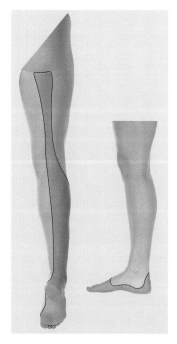

Fig. 64   The approximate area within which sensory changes may be found in lesions of both the sciatic and the posterior cutaneous nerve of the thigh.

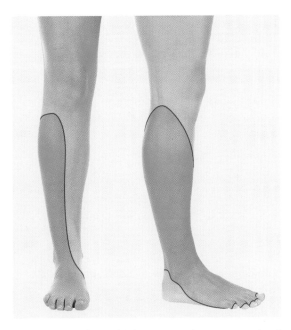

Fig. 65 The approximate area within which sensory changes may be found in lesions of the common peroneal nerve above the origin of the superficial peroneal nerve. (Modified from M.R.C. Special Report No. 54, 1920.)

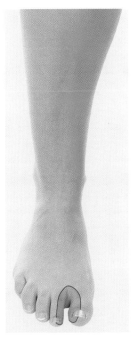

Fig. 66 The approximate area within which sensory changes may be found in lesions of the deep peroneal nerve.

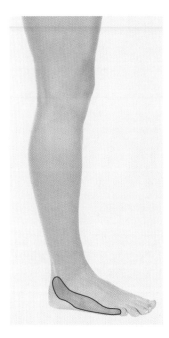

Fig. 67 The approximate area within which sensory changes may be found in lesions of the sural nerve.

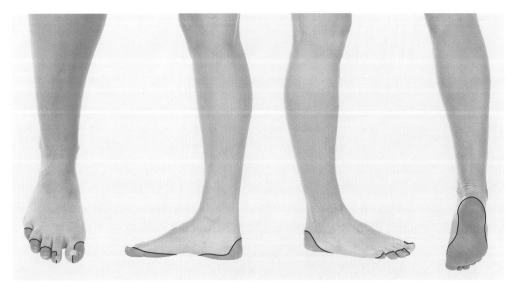

Fig. 68 The approximate area within which sensory changes may be found in lesions of the tibial nerve. (Modified from M.R.C. Special Report No. 54, 1920.)

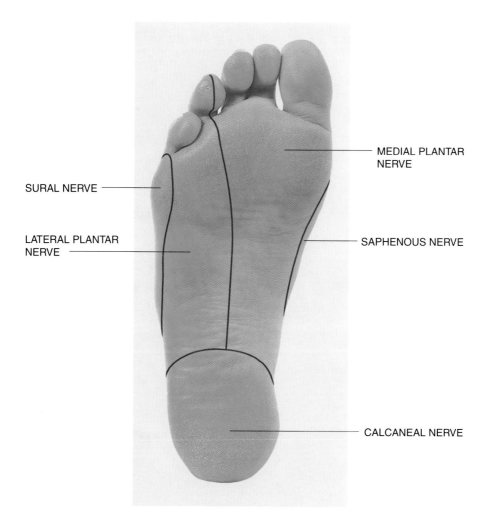

SURAL NERVE

LATERAL PLANTAR
NERVE

MEDIAL PLANTAR
NERVE

SAPHENOUS NERVE

CALCANEAL NERVE

Fig. 69   The approximate areas supplied by the cutaneous nerves to the sole of the foot.

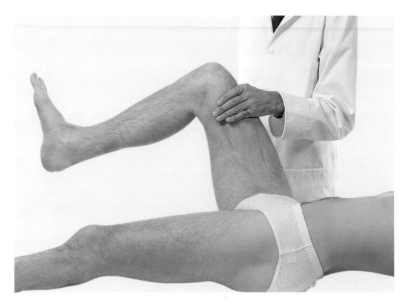

Fig. 70 Iliopsoas (Branches from L1, 2 and 3 spinal nerves and femoral nerve; **L1, L2**, L3)

The patient is flexing the thigh at the hip against resistance with the leg flexed at the knee and hip.

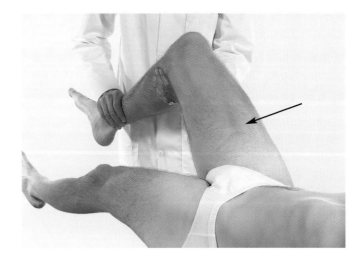

Fig. 71 Quadriceps Femoris (Femoral nerve; L2, **L3, L4**)

The patient is extending the leg against resistance with the limb flexed at the hip and knee. To detect slight weakness, the leg should be fully flexed at the knee.
Arrow: the muscle belly of rectus femoris can be seen and felt.

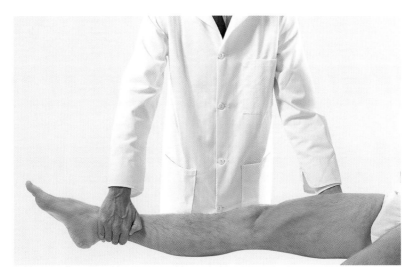

Fig. 72 Adductors (Obturator nerve; **L2**, **L3**, L4)

The patient lies on his back with the leg extended at the knee, and is adducting the limb against resistance. The muscle bellies can be felt.

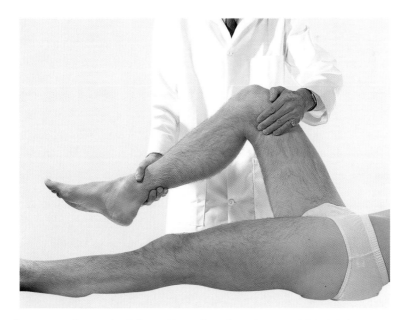

Fig. 73 Gluteus Medius and Minimus (Superior gluteal nerve; **L4**, **L5**, S1)

The patient lies on his back and is internally rotating the thigh against resistance with the limb flexed at the hip and knee.

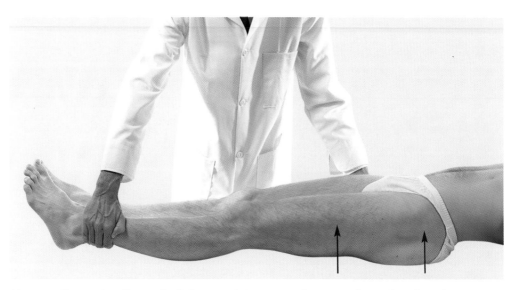

Fig. 74 Gluteus Medius and Minimus and Tensor Fasciae Latae (Superior gluteal nerve; **L4, L5**, S1)

The patient lies on his back with the leg extended and is abducting the limb against resistance. *Arrows*: the muscle bellies can be felt and sometimes seen.

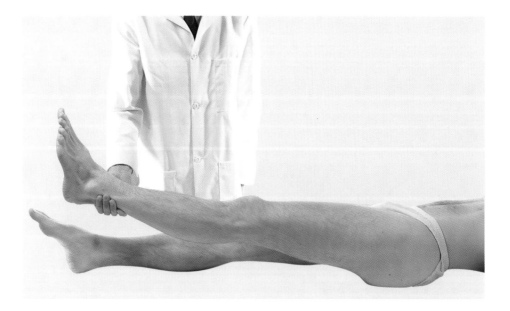

Fig. 75 Gluteus Maximus (Inferior gluteal nerve; **L5, S1**, S2)

The patient lies on his back with the leg extended at the knee and is extending the limb at the hip against resistance.

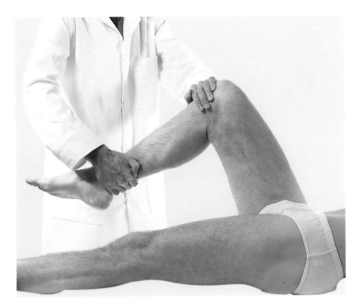

Fig. 76 Hamstring Muscles (Sciatic nerve. Semitendinosus, semimembranosus and biceps; L5, **S1**, S2)

The patient lies on his back with the limb flexed at the hip and knee and is flexing the leg at the knee against resistance.

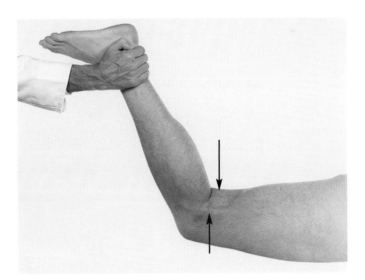

Fig. 77 Hamstring Muscles (Sciatic nerve. Semitendinosus, semimembranosus and biceps; L5, **S1**, S2)

The patient lies on his face and is flexing the leg at the knee against resistance.
Arrows: the tendons of the biceps (laterally) and semitendinosus (medially) can be felt and usually seen.

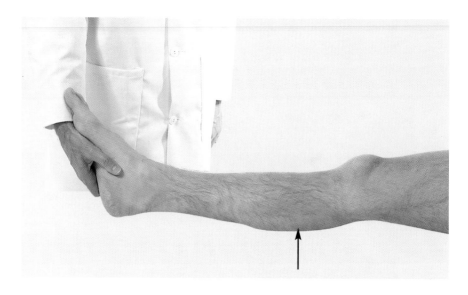

Fig. 78 Gastrocnemius (Tibial nerve; S1, S2)

The patient lies on his back with the leg extended and is plantar-flexing the foot against resistance. *Arrow*: the muscle bellies can be seen and felt. To detect slight weakness, the patient should be asked to stand on one foot, raise the heel from the ground and maintain this position.

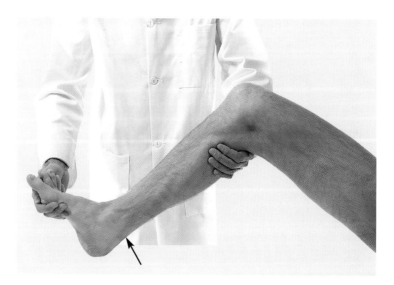

Fig. 79 Soleus (Tibial nerve; S1, S2)

The patient lies on his back with the limb flexed at the hip and knee and is plantar-flexing the foot against resistance. The muscle belly can be felt and sometimes seen.
Arrow: the Achilles tendon.

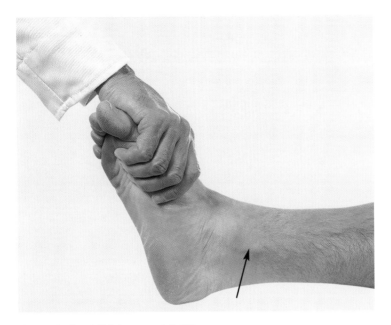

Fig. 80 Tibialis Posterior (Tibial nerve; L4, L5)

The patient is inverting the foot against resistance.
Arrow: the tendon can be seen and felt.

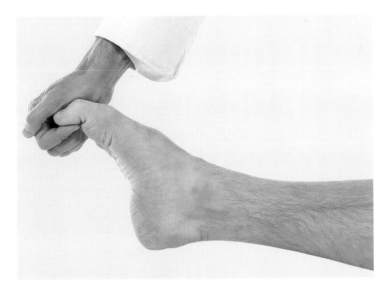

Fig. 81 Flexor Digitorum Longus, Flexor Hallucis Longus (Tibial nerve; L5, **S1, S2**)

The patient is flexing the toes against resistance.

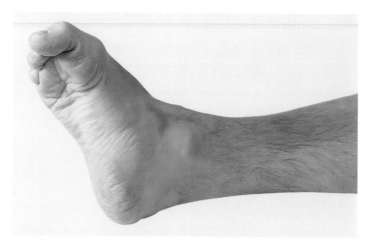

Fig. 82 Small muscles of the foot (medial and lateral plantar nerves; S1, S2)

The patient is cupping the sole of the foot; the small muscles can be felt and sometimes seen.

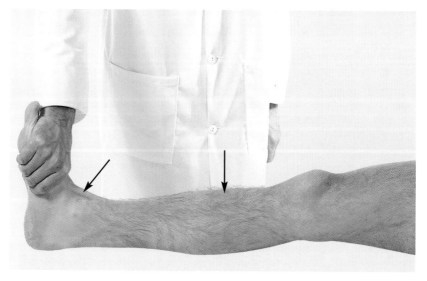

Fig. 83 Tibialis Anterior (Deep peroneal nerve; **L4**, **L5**)

The patient is dorsiflexing the foot against resistance.

Arrows: the muscle belly and its tendon can be seen and felt.

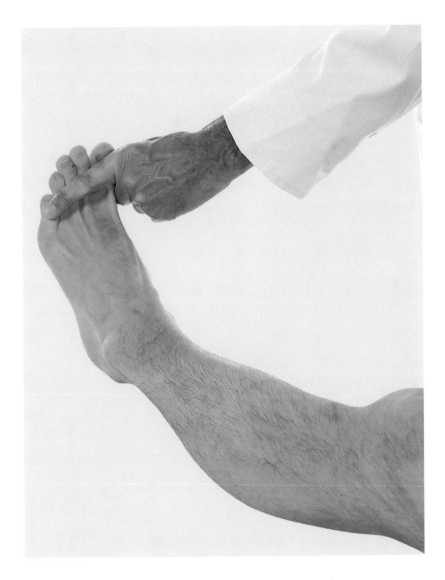

Fig. 84   Extensor Digitorum Longus (Deep peroneal nerve; **L5**, S1)

The patient is dorsiflexing the toes against resistance. The tendons passing to the lateral four toes can be seen and felt.

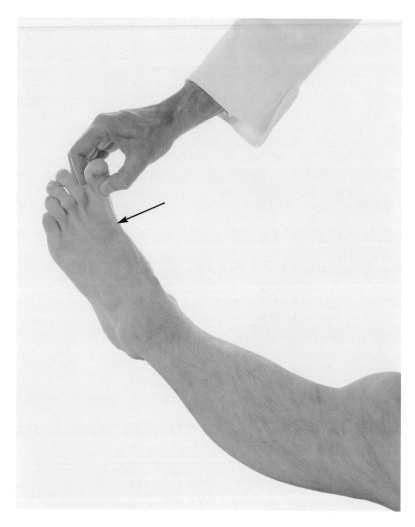

Fig. 85 Extensor Hallucis Longus (Deep peroneal nerve; **L5**, S1)

The patient is dorsiflexing the distal phalanx of the big toe against resistance. *Arrow:* the tendon can be seen and felt.

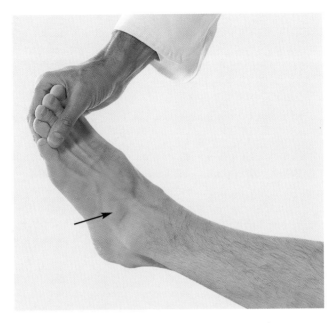

Fig. 86   Extensor Digitorum Brevis (Deep peroneal nerve; L5, S1)

The patient is dorsiflexing the proximal phalanges of the toes against resistance.
Arrow: the muscle belly can be felt and sometimes seen.

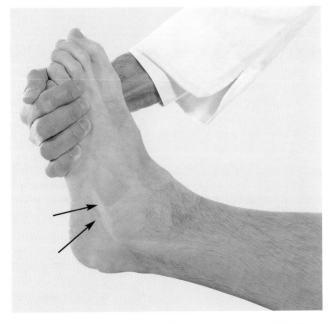

Fig. 87   Peroneus Longus and Brevis (Superficial peroneal nerve; L5, S1)

The patient is everting the foot against resistance. *Upper arrow:* the tendon of peroneus
brevis. *Lower arrow:* the tendon of peroneus longus.

DERMATOMES

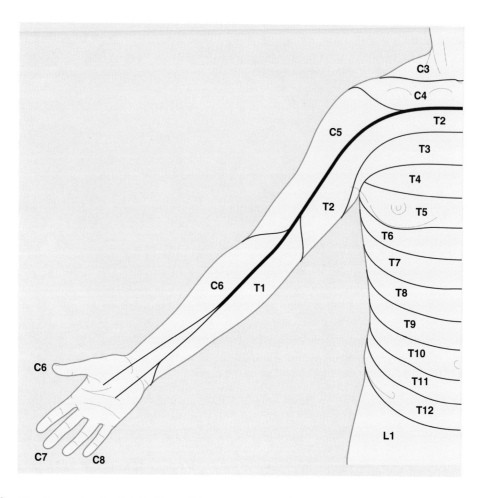

Fig. 88 Approximate distribution of dermatomes on the anterior aspect of the upper limb.

Fig. 88–91 show the approximate cutaneous areas supplied by each spinal root. There is considerable variation and overlap between dermatomes, so that an isolated root lesion results in a much smaller area of sensory impairment than is indicated in these diagrams.

This variation also applies to the innervation of the fingers, but the thumb is usually supplied by C6 and the little finger usually by C8 (see Inouye and Buchthal (1977) *Brain* **100**: 731–748).The heavy axial lines are usually more consistent, showing the boundary between non consecutive dermatomes.

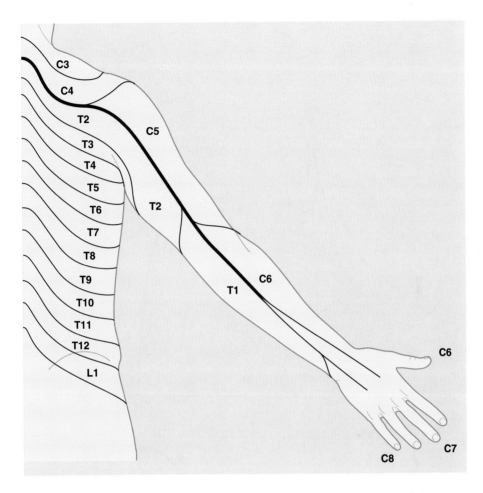

Fig. 89 Approximate distribution of dermatomes on the posterior aspect of the upper limb.

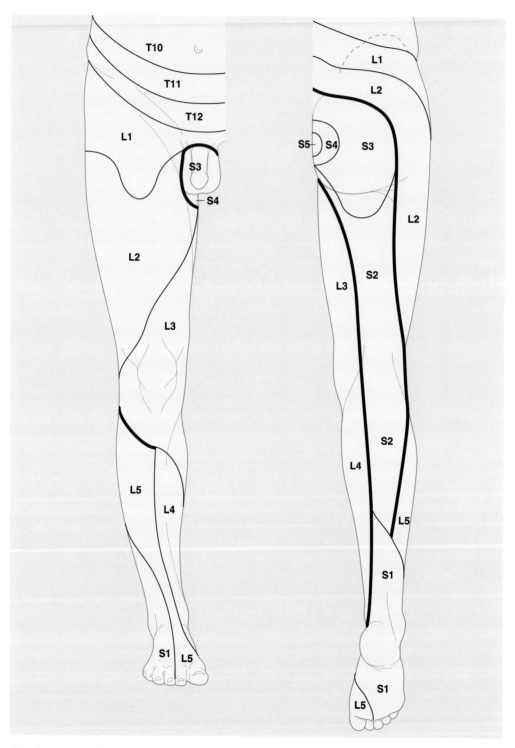

Fig. 90 Approximate distribution of dermatomes on the lower limb.

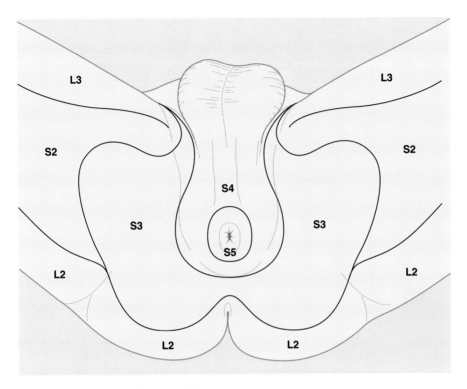

Fig. 91 Approximate distribution of dermatomes on the perineum

NERVES AND MAIN ROOT SUPPLY OF MUSCLES

The list given below does not include all the muscles innervated by these nerves, but only those more commonly tested, either clinically or electrically, and shows the order of innervation.

Upper Limb	Spinal Roots
Spinal Accessory Nerve	
Trapezius	C3, C4
Brachial Plexus	
Rhomboids	C4, C5
Serratus anterior	C5, C6, C7
Pectoralis major	
Clavicular ⎤	**C5**, C6
Sternal ⎦	C6, **C7**, C8
Supraspinatus	**C5**, C6
Infraspinatus	**C5**, C6
Latissimus dorsi	C6, **C7**, C8
Teres major	C5, C6, C7
Axillary Nerve	
Deltoid	**C5**, C6
Musculocutaneous Nerve	
Biceps	C5, C6
Brachialis	C5, C6
Radial Nerve	
Triceps ⎰ Long head ⎱	
⎱ Lateral head ⎰	C6, **C7**, C8
⎱ Medial head ⎰	
Brachioradialis	C5, **C6**
Extensor carpi radialis longus	C5, **C6**
Posterior Interosseous Nerve	
Supinator	C6, C7
Extensor carpi ulnaris	**C7**, C8
Extensor digitorum	**C7**, C8
Abductor pollicis longus	**C7**, C8
Extensor pollicis longus	**C7**, C8
Extensor pollicis brevis	**C7**, C8
Extensor indicis	**C7**, C8
Median Nerve	
Pronator teres	C6, C7
Flexor carpi radialis	C6, C7
Flexor digitorum superficialis	C7, **C8**, T1
Abductor pollicis brevis	C8, **T1**
Flexor pollicis brevis*	C8, **T1**
Opponens pollicis	C8, **T1**
Lumbricals I & II	C8, **T1**

Anterior Interosseous Nerve
Pronator quadratus   C7, **C8**
Flexor digitorum profundus I & II   C7, **C8**
Flexor pollicis longus   C7, **C8**

Ulnar Nerve
Flexor carpi ulnaris   C7, **C8**, T1
Flexor digitorum profundus III & IV   C7, **C8**
Hypothenar muscles   **C8, T1**
Adductor pollicis   **C8, T1**
Flexor pollicis brevis   **C8, T1**
Palmar interossei   **C8, T1**
Dorsal interossei   **C8, T1**
Lumbricals III & IV   **C8, T1**

Lower Limb	**Spinal Roots**

Femoral Nerve
Iliopsoas   **L1, L2,** L3

Rectus femoris ⎫
Vastus lateralis ⎬ Quadriceps   L2, **L3, L4**
Vastus intermedius ⎪ femoris
Vastus medialis ⎭

Obturator Nerve
Adductor longus ⎫   **L2, L3,** L4
Adductor magnus ⎭

Superior Gluteal Nerve
Gluteus medus and minimus ⎫   **L4, L5,** S1
Tensor fasciae latae ⎭

Inferior Gluteal Nerve
Gluteus maximus   **L5, S1,** S2

Sciatic and Tibial Nerves
Semitendinosus   **L5, S1,** S2
Biceps   **L5, S1,** S2
Semimembranosus   **L5, S1,** S2
Gastrocnemius and soleus   S1, S2
Tibialis posterior   L4, L5
Flexor digitorum longus   **L5, S1, S2**
Abductor hallucis ⎫
Abductor digiti minimi ⎬ Small muscles   S1, S2
Interossei ⎭ of foot

Sciatic and Common Peroneal Nerves
Tibialis anterior   **L4,** L5
Extensor digitorum longus   **L5,** S1
Extensor hallucis longus   **L5,** S1
Extensor digitorum brevis   L5, S1
Peroneus longus   L5, S1
Peroneus brevis   L5, S1

*Flexor pollicis brevis is often supplied wholly or partially by the ulnar nerve.

COMMONLY TESTED MOVEMENTS

Movement	UMN	Root	Reflex	Nerve	Muscle
Upper limb					
Shoulder abduction	++	C5		Axillary	Deltoid
Elbow flexion		C5/6	+	Musculocutaneous	Biceps
		C6	+	Radial	Brachioradialis
Elbow extension	+	C7	+	Radial	Triceps
Radial wrist extension	+	C6		Radial	Extensor carpi radialis longus
Finger extension	+	C7		Posterior interosseus nerve	Extensor digitorum communis
Finger flexion		C8	+	Anterior interosseus nerve	Flexor pollicis longus + Flexor digitorum profundus (index)
				Ulnar	Flexor digitorum profundus (ring + little)
Finger abduction	++	T1		Ulnar	First dorsal interosseous
		T1		Median	Abductor pollicis brevis
Lower limb					
Hip flexion	++	L1/2			Iliopsoas
Hip adduction		L2/3	+	Obturator	Adductors
Hip extension		L5/S1		Sciatic	Gluteus maximus
Knee flexion	+	S1		Sciatic	Hamstrings
Knee extension		L3/4	+	Femoral	Quadriceps
Ankle dorsiflexion	++	L4		Deep peroneal	Tibialis anterior
Ankle eversion		L5/S1		Superficial peroneal	Peronei
Ankle plantarflexion		S1/S2	+	Tibial	Gastrocnemius, soleus
Big toe extension		L5		Deep peroneal	Extensor hallucis longus

The table shows some commonly tested movements, the principal muscle involved with its roots and nerve supply. The column headed UMN indicates those movements which are preferentially weak in upper motor neuron lesions.